There is a saying - you can't

manage

what you don't measure.

Measuring your intake helps you

manage your output.

A healthier inside makes for a

more attractive outside.

Become your own Boss today, by managing what you eat, and how you use those calories

Notes:

Mahatma Gandhi

Your beliefs become your thoughts,
Your thoughts become your words,
Your words become your actions,
Your actions become your habits,
Your habits become your values,
Your values become your destiny.

Notes:

My Habit Tracker

Becoming aware of your actions helps to make sure you are taking the right ones.

Negative Habit	Why is it a negative habit?	What steps can I take to change it?

Notes:

Habit Tracker

Month _____

Year _____

Day													
1													
2													
3													
4													
5													
6													
7													
8													
9													
10													
11													
12													
13													
14													
15													
16													
17													
18													
19													
20													
21													
22													
23													
24													
25													
26													
27													
28													
29													
30													
31													

Notes:

Don't let what you didn't do today get in the way of you can do tomorrow!

Date:

6 am	
7	
8	
9	
10	
11	
12 pm	
1	
2	
3	
4	
5	
6	
7	
8	

Notes:_____

_____

_____

_____

To Do

Happiness

100%

75% 45%

60%

Accomplishments

☐ . . . .
☐ . . . .
☐ . . . .
☐ . . . .

Date		S M T W T F S	
Breakfast	Amount	Calories (kcal)	
	Total		
Snack	Amount	Calories (kcal)	
	Total		
Lunch	Amount	Calories (kcal)	
	Total		

Snack	Amount	Calories (kcal)
	Total	
Dinner	Amount	Calories (kcal)
	Total	
Snack	Amount	Calories (kcal)
	Total	
Exercise	Duration	Calories burned (kcal)

Water									Fruit & Veggies							

Notes:

Don't rush the process, consistence delivers results!

Date:

6 am	
7	
8	
9	
10	
11	
12 pm	
1	
2	
3	
4	
5	
6	
7	
8	

To Do

Happiness

100%

75%   45%

60%

Accomplishments

☐ . . . .
☐ . . . .
☐ . . . .
☐ . . . .

Notes:_____

_____

_____

_____

Date	S M T W T F S	
Breakfast	Amount	Calories (kcal)
	Total	
Snack	Amount	Calories (kcal)
	Total	
Lunch	Amount	Calories (kcal)
	Total	

Snack	Amount	Calories (kcal)
	Total	
Dinner	Amount	Calories (kcal)
	Total	
Snack	Amount	Calories (kcal)
	Total	
Exercise	Duration	Calories burned (kcal)
Water	Fruit & Veggies	

Notes:

Don't let what you didn't do today get in the way of you can do tomorrow!

Date:

| 6 am |
| 7 |
| 8 |
| 9 |
| 10 |
| 11 |
| 12 pm |
| 1 |
| 2 |
| 3 |
| 4 |
| 5 |
| 6 |
| 7 |
| 8 |

Notes:_____

_____

_____

_____

To Do

Happiness

100%

75% 45%

60%

Accomplishments

☐ . . . .
☐ . . . .
☐ . . . .
☐ . . . .

Date		S M T W T F S
Breakfast	Amount	Calories (kcal)
	Total	
Snack	Amount	Calories (kcal)
	Total	
Lunch	Amount	Calories (kcal)
	Total	

Snack	Amount	Calories (kcal)
	Total	
Dinner	Amount	Calories (kcal)
	Total	
Snack	Amount	Calories (kcal)
	Total	
Exercise	Duration	Calories burned (kcal)
Water		Fruit & Veggies

Notes:

Don't rush the process, consistence delivers results!

Date:

Time	
6 am	
7	
8	
9	
10	
11	
12 pm	
1	
2	
3	
4	
5	
6	
7	
8	

Notes:_____

_____

_____

_____

To Do

Happiness

100%

75%   45%

60%

Accomplishments

- [ ] . . . .
- [ ] . . . .
- [ ] . . . .
- [ ] . . . .

Date		S M T W T F S
Breakfast	Amount	Calories (kcal)
	Total	
Snack	Amount	Calories (kcal)
	Total	
Lunch	Amount	Calories (kcal)
	Total	

Snack	Amount	Calories (kcal)
	Total	
Dinner	Amount	Calories (kcal)
	Total	
Snack	Amount	Calories (kcal)
	Total	
Exercise	Duration	Calories burned (kcal)
Water		Fruit & Veggies	

Notes:

Don't let what you didn't do today get in the way of you can do tomorrow!

Date:

6 am
7
8
9
10
11
12 pm
1
2
3
4
5
6
7
8

Notes:_____

_____

_____

_____

To Do

Happiness

100%

75%   45%

60%

Accomplishments

☐. . . . .

☐. . . . .

☐. . . . .

☐. . . . .

Date		S M T W T F S	
Breakfast		Amount	Calories (kcal)
		Total	
Snack		Amount	Calories (kcal)
		Total	
Lunch		Amount	Calories (kcal)
		Total	

Snack	Amount	Calories (kcal)
	Total	
Dinner	Amount	Calories (kcal)
	Total	
Snack	Amount	Calories (kcal)
	Total	
Exercise	Duration	Calories burned (kcal)
Water		Fruit & Veggies	

Notes:

Don't rush the process, consistence delivers results!

Date:

Time	
6 am	
7	
8	
9	
10	
11	
12 pm	
1	
2	
3	
4	
5	
6	
7	
8	

To Do

Happiness

100%

75%   45%

60%

Accomplishments

☐ . . . .
☐ . . . .
☐ . . . .
☐ . . . .

Notes:_____
_____
_____
_____

Date		S M T W T F S	
Breakfast		Amount	Calories (kcal)
		Total	
Snack		Amount	Calories (kcal)
		Total	
Lunch		Amount	Calories (kcal)
		Total	

Snack	Amount	Calories (kcal)
	Total	
Dinner	Amount	Calories (kcal)
	Total	
Snack	Amount	Calories (kcal)
	Total	
Exercise	Duration	Calories burned (kcal)
Water									Fruit & Veggies								

Notes:

Don't let what you didn't do today get in the way of you can do tomorrow!

Date:

| 6 am |
| 7 |
| 8 |
| 9 |
| 10 |
| 11 |
| 12 pm |
| 1 |
| 2 |
| 3 |
| 4 |
| 5 |
| 6 |
| 7 |
| 8 |

Notes:_____

_____

_____

_____

To Do

Happiness

100%

75% 45%

60%

Accomplishments

☐ . . . .
☐ . . . .
☐ . . . .
☐ . . . .

Date	S M T W T F S	
Breakfast	Amount	Calories (kcal)
	Total	
Snack	Amount	Calories (kcal)
	Total	
Lunch	Amount	Calories (kcal)
	Total	

Snack	Amount	Calories (kcal)
	Total	
Dinner	Amount	Calories (kcal)
	Total	
Snack	Amount	Calories (kcal)
	Total	
Exercise	Duration	Calories burned (kcal)
Water		Fruit & Veggies	

Notes:

Don't rush the process, consistence delivers results!

Date:

Time	
6 am	
7	
8	
9	
10	
11	
12 pm	
1	
2	
3	
4	
5	
6	
7	
8	

Notes:_____

_____

_____

_____

To Do

Happiness

100%

75%   45%

60%

Accomplishments

☐ . . . .

☐ . . . .

☐ . . . .

☐ . . . .

Date	S M T W T F S	
Breakfast	Amount	Calories (kcal)
	Total	
Snack	Amount	Calories (kcal)
	Total	
Lunch	Amount	Calories (kcal)
	Total	

Snack	Amount	Calories (kcal)
	Total	
Dinner	Amount	Calories (kcal)
	Total	
Snack	Amount	Calories (kcal)
	Total	
Exercise	Duration	Calories burned (kcal)
Water		Fruit & Veggies	

Notes:

Don't let what you didn't do today get in the way of you can do tomorrow!

Date:

	To Do
6 am	
7	
8	
9	
10	
11	
12 pm	

Happiness

100%

75% 45%

60%

Accomplishments

1	
2	
3	
4	
5	
6	
7	
8	

Notes:_____

_____

_____

_____

Date		S M T W T F S
Breakfast	Amount	Calories (kcal)
	Total	
Snack	Amount	Calories (kcal)
	Total	
Lunch	Amount	Calories (kcal)
	Total	

Snack	Amount	Calories (kcal)
	Total	
Dinner	Amount	Calories (kcal)
	Total	
Snack	Amount	Calories (kcal)
	Total	
Exercise	Duration	Calories burned (kcal)
Water		Fruit & Veggies	

Notes:

Don't rush the process, consistence delivers results!

Date:

Time	
6 am	
7	
8	
9	
10	
11	
12 pm	
1	
2	
3	
4	
5	
6	
7	
8	

Notes:_____

_____

_____

_____

To Do

Happiness

100%

75%   45%

60%

Accomplishments

- . . . .
- . . . .
- . . . .
- . . . .

Date		S M T W T F S	
Breakfast		Amount	Calories (kcal)
		Total	
Snack		Amount	Calories (kcal)
		Total	
Lunch		Amount	Calories (kcal)
		Total	

Snack	Amount	Calories (kcal)
	Total	
Dinner	Amount	Calories (kcal)
	Total	
Snack	Amount	Calories (kcal)
	Total	
Exercise	Duration	Calories burned (kcal)
Water		Fruit & Veggies

Notes:

Don't let what you didn't do today get in the way of you can do tomorrow!

Date:

6 am	
7	
8	
9	
10	
11	
12 pm	
1	
2	
3	
4	
5	
6	
7	
8	

Notes:_____

_____

_____

_____

To Do

Happiness

100%

75%   45%

60%

Accomplishments

☐ . . . .

☐ . . . .

☐ . . . .

☐ . . . .

Date		S M T W T F S	
Breakfast		Amount	Calories (kcal)
		Total	
Snack		Amount	Calories (kcal)
		Total	
Lunch		Amount	Calories (kcal)
		Total	

Snack	Amount	Calories (kcal)
	Total	
Dinner	Amount	Calories (kcal)
	Total	
Snack	Amount	Calories (kcal)
	Total	
Exercise	Duration	Calories burned (kcal)
Water		Fruit & Veggies	

Notes:

Don't rush the process, consistence delivers results!

Date:

Time	
6 am	
7	
8	
9	
10	
11	
12 pm	
1	
2	
3	
4	
5	
6	
7	
8	

To Do

Happiness

100%

75%   45%

60%

Accomplishments

☐ . . . .

☐ . . . .

☐ . . . .

☐ . . . .

Notes:_____

_____

_____

_____

Date		S M T W T F S	
Breakfast	Amount	Calories (kcal)	
	Total		
Snack	Amount	Calories (kcal)	
	Total		
Lunch	Amount	Calories (kcal)	
	Total		

Snack	Amount	Calories (kcal)
	Total	
Dinner	Amount	Calories (kcal)
	Total	
Snack	Amount	Calories (kcal)
	Total	
Exercise	Duration	Calories burned (kcal)

Water									Fruit & Veggies								

Notes:

Don't let what you didn't do today get in the way of you can do tomorrow!

Date:

Time	
6 am	
7	
8	
9	
10	
11	
12 pm	
1	
2	
3	
4	
5	
6	
7	
8	

Notes:_____

_____

_____

_____

To Do

Happiness

100%

75%   45%

60%

Accomplishments

☐. . . . .

☐. . . . .

☐. . . . .

☐. . . . .

Date		S M T W T F S	
Breakfast		Amount	Calories (kcal)
		Total	
Snack		Amount	Calories (kcal)
		Total	
Lunch		Amount	Calories (kcal)
		Total	

Snack	Amount	Calories (kcal)
	Total	
Dinner	Amount	Calories (kcal)
	Total	
Snack	Amount	Calories (kcal)
	Total	
Exercise	Duration	Calories burned (kcal)
Water									Fruit & Veggies								

Notes:

Don't rush the process, consistence delivers results!

Date:

Time	
6 am	
7	
8	
9	
10	
11	
12 pm	
1	
2	
3	
4	
5	
6	
7	
8	

To Do

Happiness

100%

75%   45%

60%

Accomplishments

☐ . . . .
☐ . . . .
☐ . . . .
☐ . . . .

Notes:_____
_____
_____
_____

Date		S M T W T F S	
Breakfast		Amount	Calories (kcal)
		Total	
Snack		Amount	Calories (kcal)
		Total	
Lunch		Amount	Calories (kcal)
		Total	

Snack	Amount	Calories (kcal)
	Total	
Dinner	Amount	Calories (kcal)
	Total	
Snack	Amount	Calories (kcal)
	Total	
Exercise	Duration	Calories burned (kcal)

Water									Fruit & Veggies							

Notes:

Don't let what you didn't do today get in the way of you can do tomorrow!

Date:

6 am	**To Do**
7	
8	
9	
10	
11	
12 pm	
1	**Happiness**
2	100%
3	75% 45%
4	60%
5	
6	
7	**Accomplishments**
8	

Notes:_____

_____

_____

_____

- [ ] . . . .
- [ ] . . . .
- [ ] . . . .
- [ ] . . . .

Date		S M T W T F S	
Breakfast		Amount	Calories (kcal)
		Total	
Snack		Amount	Calories (kcal)
		Total	
Lunch		Amount	Calories (kcal)
		Total	

Snack	Amount	Calories (kcal)
	Total	
Dinner	Amount	Calories (kcal)
	Total	
Snack	Amount	Calories (kcal)
	Total	
Exercise	Duration	Calories burned (kcal)
Water		Fruit & Veggies	

Notes:

Don't rush the process, consistence delivers results!

Date:

Time	
6 am	
7	
8	
9	
10	
11	
12 pm	
1	
2	
3	
4	
5	
6	
7	
8	

To Do

Happiness

100%

75%   45%

60%

Accomplishments

☐ . . . .
☐ . . . .
☐ . . . .
☐ . . . .

Notes:_____

_____

_____

_____

Date	S M T W T F S	
Breakfast	Amount	Calories (kcal)
	Total	
Snack	Amount	Calories (kcal)
	Total	
Lunch	Amount	Calories (kcal)
	Total	

Snack	Amount	Calories (kcal)
	Total	
Dinner	Amount	Calories (kcal)
	Total	
Snack	Amount	Calories (kcal)
	Total	
Exercise	Duration	Calories burned (kcal)

Water									Fruit & Veggies							

Notes:

Don't let what you didn't do today get in the way of you can do tomorrow!

Date:

6 am	
7	
8	
9	
10	
11	
12 pm	
1	
2	
3	
4	
5	
6	
7	
8	

Notes:_____

_____

_____

_____

To Do

Happiness

100%

75%   45%

60%

Accomplishments

☐ . . . .

☐ . . . .

☐ . . . .

☐ . . . .

Date	S M T W T F S	
Breakfast	Amount	Calories (kcal)
	Total	
Snack	Amount	Calories (kcal)
	Total	
Lunch	Amount	Calories (kcal)
	Total	

Snack	Amount	Calories (kcal)
	Total	
Dinner	Amount	Calories (kcal)
	Total	
Snack	Amount	Calories (kcal)
	Total	
Exercise	Duration	Calories burned (kcal)
Water									Fruit & Veggies							

Notes:

Don't rush the process, consistence delivers results!

Date:

6 am

7

8

9

10

11

12 pm

1

2

3

4

5

6

7

8

To Do

Happiness

100%

75%   45%

60%

Accomplishments

- [ ] . . . .
- [ ] . . . .
- [ ] . . . .
- [ ] . . . .

Notes:_____

_____

_____

_____

Date		S M T W T F S	
Breakfast	Amount	Calories (kcal)	
	Total		
Snack	Amount	Calories (kcal)	
	Total		
Lunch	Amount	Calories (kcal)	
	Total		

Snack	Amount	Calories (kcal)
	Total	
Dinner	Amount	Calories (kcal)
	Total	
Snack	Amount	Calories (kcal)
	Total	
Exercise	Duration	Calories burned (kcal)
Water		Fruit & Veggies	

Notes:

Don't let what you didn't do today get in the way of you can do tomorrow!

Date:

Time	
6 am	
7	
8	
9	
10	
11	
12 pm	
1	
2	
3	
4	
5	
6	
7	
8	

Notes:_____

_____

_____

_____

To Do

Happiness

100%

75%   45%

60%

Accomplishments

☐. . . . .

☐. . . . .

☐. . . . .

☐. . . . .

Date		S M T W T F S	
Breakfast		Amount	Calories (kcal)
		Total	
Snack		Amount	Calories (kcal)
		Total	
Lunch		Amount	Calories (kcal)
		Total	

Snack	Amount	Calories (kcal)
	Total	
Dinner	Amount	Calories (kcal)
	Total	
Snack	Amount	Calories (kcal)
	Total	
Exercise	Duration	Calories burned (kcal)
Water		Fruit & Veggies		

Notes:

Don't rush the process, consistence delivers results!

Date:

Time	
6 am	
7	
8	
9	
10	
11	
12 pm	
1	
2	
3	
4	
5	
6	
7	
8	

To Do

Happiness

100%

75% 45%

60%

Accomplishments

☐ . . . .
☐ . . . .
☐ . . . .
☐ . . . .

Notes:_____

_____

_____

_____

Date		S M T W T F S	
Breakfast		Amount	Calories (kcal)
		Total	
Snack		Amount	Calories (kcal)
		Total	
Lunch		Amount	Calories (kcal)
		Total	

Snack	Amount	Calories (kcal)
	Total	
Dinner	Amount	Calories (kcal)
	Total	
Snack	Amount	Calories (kcal)
	Total	
Exercise	Duration	Calories burned (kcal)
Water		Fruit & Veggies	

Notes:

Don't let what you didn't do today get in the way of you can do tomorrow!

6 am

7

8

9

10

11

12 pm

1

2

3

4

5

6

7

8

To Do

Happiness

100%

75% 45%

60%

Accomplishments

☐. . . . .

☐. . . . .

☐. . . . .

☐. . . . .

Notes:_____

_____

_____

_____

Date		S M T W T F S	
Breakfast		Amount	Calories (kcal)
		Total	
Snack		Amount	Calories (kcal)
		Total	
Lunch		Amount	Calories (kcal)
		Total	

Snack	Amount	Calories (kcal)
	Total	
Dinner	Amount	Calories (kcal)
	Total	
Snack	Amount	Calories (kcal)
	Total	
Exercise	Duration	Calories burned (kcal)
Water		Fruit & Veggies	

Notes:

Don't rush the process, consistence delivers results!

Date:

Time	
6 am	
7	
8	
9	
10	
11	
12 pm	
1	
2	
3	
4	
5	
6	
7	
8	

Notes: _____

_____

_____

_____

To Do

Happiness

100%

75%   45%

60%

Accomplishments

☐ . . . .

☐ . . . .

☐ . . . .

☐ . . . .

Date		S M T W T F S	
Breakfast		Amount	Calories (kcal)
		Total	
Snack		Amount	Calories (kcal)
		Total	
Lunch		Amount	Calories (kcal)
		Total	

Snack	Amount	Calories (kcal)
	Total	
Dinner	Amount	Calories (kcal)
	Total	
Snack	Amount	Calories (kcal)
	Total	
Exercise	Duration	Calories burned (kcal)

Water								Fruit & Veggies							

Notes:

Don't let what you didn't do today get in the way of you can do tomorrow!

Date:

6 am	
7	
8	
9	
10	
11	
12 pm	
1	
2	
3	
4	
5	
6	
7	
8	

Notes:_____

_____

_____

_____

To Do

Happiness

100%

75%   45%

60%

Accomplishments

☐ . . . .

☐ . . . .

☐ . . . .

☐ . . . .

Date	S M T W T F S	
Breakfast	Amount	Calories (kcal)
	Total	
Snack	Amount	Calories (kcal)
	Total	
Lunch	Amount	Calories (kcal)
	Total	

Snack	Amount	Calories (kcal)
	Total	
Dinner	Amount	Calories (kcal)
	Total	
Snack	Amount	Calories (kcal)
	Total	
Exercise	Duration	Calories burned (kcal)
Water		Fruit & Veggies	

Notes:

Don't rush the process, consistence delivers results!

Date:

Time	
6 am	
7	
8	
9	
10	
11	
12 pm	
1	
2	
3	
4	
5	
6	
7	
8	

To Do

Happiness

100%

75%   45%

60%

Accomplishments

- [ ]
- [ ]
- [ ]
- [ ]

Notes:_____

_____

_____

_____

Date		S M T W T F S	
Breakfast		Amount	Calories (kcal)
		Total	
Snack		Amount	Calories (kcal)
		Total	
Lunch		Amount	Calories (kcal)
		Total	

Snack	Amount	Calories (kcal)
	Total	
Dinner	Amount	Calories (kcal)
	Total	
Snack	Amount	Calories (kcal)
	Total	
Exercise	Duration	Calories burned (kcal)
Water	Fruit & Veggies	

Notes:

Don't let what you didn't do today get in the way of you can do tomorrow!

Date:

6 am	
7	**To Do**
8	
9	
10	
11	
12 pm	
1	**Happiness**
2	
3	100%
4	75% 45%
5	60%
6	
7	**Accomplishments**
8	

Notes:_____

_____

_____

_____

☐ . . . .

☐ . . . .

☐ . . . .

☐ . . . .

Date		S M T W T F S	
Breakfast		Amount	Calories (kcal)
		Total	
Snack		Amount	Calories (kcal)
		Total	
Lunch		Amount	Calories (kcal)
		Total	

Snack	Amount	Calories (kcal)
	Total	
Dinner	Amount	Calories (kcal)
	Total	
Snack	Amount	Calories (kcal)
	Total	
Exercise	Duration	Calories burned (kcal)

Water									Fruit & Veggies							

Notes:

Don't rush the process, consistence delivers results!

Date:

Time	
6 am	
7	
8	
9	
10	
11	
12 pm	
1	
2	
3	
4	
5	
6	
7	
8	

To Do

Happiness

100%
75% 45%
60%

Accomplishments
- ☐ . . . .
- ☐ . . . .
- ☐ . . . .
- ☐ . . . .

Notes:_____
_____
_____
_____

Date		S M T W T F S	
Breakfast		Amount	Calories (kcal)
		Total	
Snack		Amount	Calories (kcal)
		Total	
Lunch		Amount	Calories (kcal)
		Total	

Snack	Amount	Calories (kcal)
	Total	
Dinner	Amount	Calories (kcal)
	Total	
Snack	Amount	Calories (kcal)
	Total	
Exercise	Duration	Calories burned (kcal)

Water								Fruit & Veggies						

Notes:

Don't let what you didn't do today get in the way of you can do tomorrow!

Date:

| 6 am |
| 7 |
| 8 |
| 9 |
| 10 |
| 11 |
| 12 pm |
| 1 |
| 2 |
| 3 |
| 4 |
| 5 |
| 6 |
| 7 |
| 8 |

Notes:_____

_____

_____

_____

To Do

Happiness

100%

75%   45%

60%

Accomplishments

☐. . . . .
☐. . . . .
☐. . . . .
☐. . . . .

Date		S M T W T F S	
Breakfast		Amount	Calories (kcal)
		Total	
Snack		Amount	Calories (kcal)
		Total	
Lunch		Amount	Calories (kcal)
		Total	

Snack	Amount	Calories (kcal)
	Total	
Dinner	Amount	Calories (kcal)
	Total	
Snack	Amount	Calories (kcal)
	Total	
Exercise	Duration	Calories burned (kcal)
Water	Fruit & Veggies	

Notes:

Don't rush the process, consistence delivers results!

Date:

Time	
6 am	
7	
8	
9	
10	
11	
12 pm	
1	
2	
3	
4	
5	
6	
7	
8	

To Do

Happiness

100%

75%   45%

60%

Accomplishments

☐ . . . .
☐ . . . .
☐ . . . .
☐ . . . .

Notes:_____

_____

_____

_____

Date		S M T W T F S	
Breakfast		Amount	Calories (kcal)
		Total	
Snack		Amount	Calories (kcal)
		Total	
Lunch		Amount	Calories (kcal)
		Total	

Snack	Amount	Calories (kcal)
	Total	
Dinner	Amount	Calories (kcal)
	Total	
Snack	Amount	Calories (kcal)
	Total	
Exercise	Duration	Calories burned (kcal)
Water		Fruit & Veggies	

Notes:

Don't let what you didn't do today get in the way of you can do tomorrow!

Date:

6 am	
7	
8	
9	
10	
11	
12 pm	
1	
2	
3	
4	
5	
6	
7	
8	

To Do

Happiness

100%

75% 45%

60%

Accomplishments

☐. . . . .

☐. . . . .

☐. . . . .

☐. . . . .

Notes:_____

_____

_____

_____

Date	S M T W T F S	
Breakfast	Amount	Calories (kcal)
	Total	
Snack	Amount	Calories (kcal)
	Total	
Lunch	Amount	Calories (kcal)
	Total	

Snack	Amount	Calories (kcal)
	Total	
Dinner	Amount	Calories (kcal)
	Total	
Snack	Amount	Calories (kcal)
	Total	
Exercise	Duration	Calories burned (kcal)

Water									Fruit & Veggies								

Notes:

Don't rush the process, consistence delivers results!

Date:

Time	
6 am	
7	
8	
9	
10	
11	
12 pm	
1	
2	
3	
4	
5	
6	
7	
8	

To Do

Happiness

100%

75%   45%

60%

Accomplishments

☐ . . . .
☐ . . . .
☐ . . . .
☐ . . . .

Notes:_____

_____

_____

_____

Date	S M T W T F S	
Breakfast	Amount	Calories (kcal)
	Total	
Snack	Amount	Calories (kcal)
	Total	
Lunch	Amount	Calories (kcal)
	Total	

Snack	Amount	Calories (kcal)
	Total	
Dinner	Amount	Calories (kcal)
	Total	
Snack	Amount	Calories (kcal)
	Total	
Exercise	Duration	Calories burned (kcal)
Water		Fruit & Veggies	

Notes:

www.ingramcontent.com/pod-product-compliance
Lightning Source LLC
Chambersburg PA
CBHW072053280526
45788CB00006B/2279